AEROBICS
FITNESS GUIDE FOR
BEGINNERS

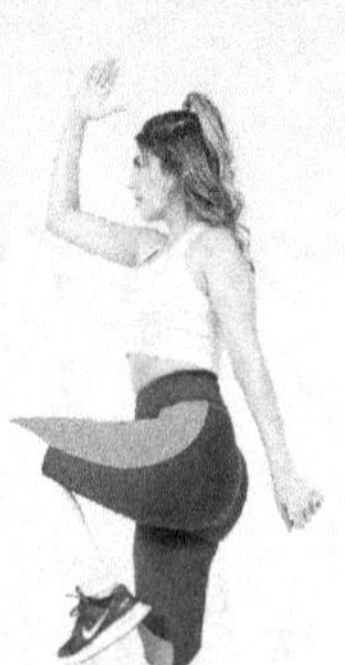

Embark on a Path of Vitality Through Active
Physical Routines

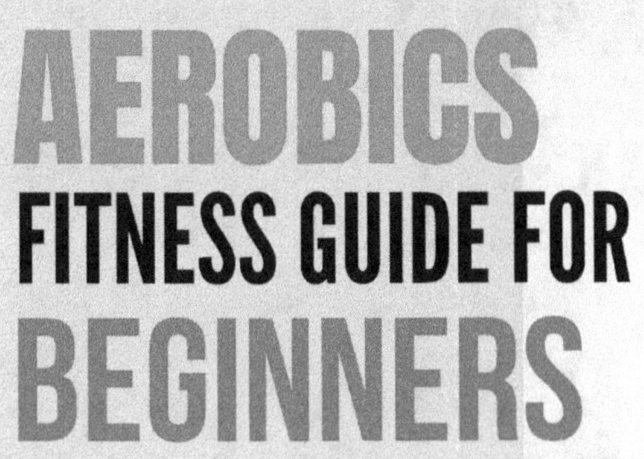

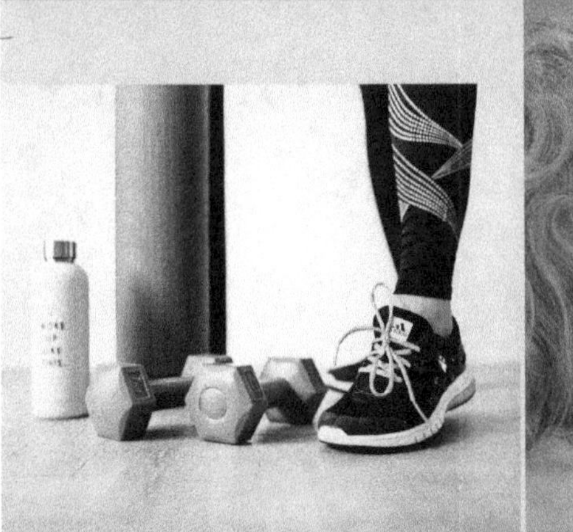

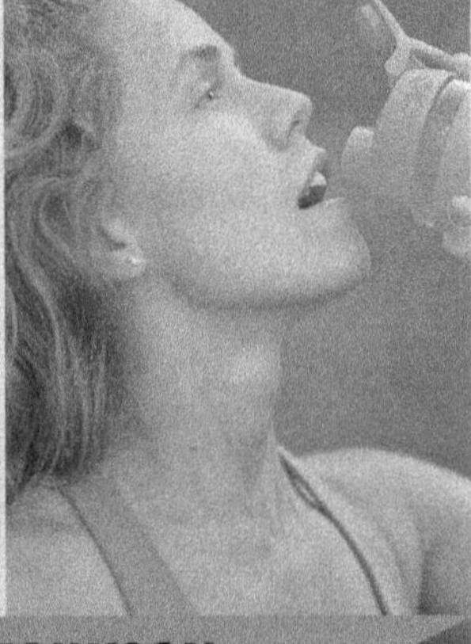

DR EDWARD A. JOHNSON

AEROBICS FITNESS GUIDE FOR BEGINNERS

Embark on a Path of Vitality Through Active Physical Routines

Dr Edward A. Johnson

Copyright © Dr. Edward A. Johnson 2023. All rights reserved.

Before this document is duplicated or reproduced in any manner, the publisher's consent must be gained. Therefore, the contents within can neither be stored electronically, transferred, nor kept in a database.

Neither in part nor full can the document be copied, scanned, faxed or retained without approval from the publisher or creator.

Table of contents

Introduction

Welcome to "Aerobics Fitness Guide for Beginners," a comprehensive guide designed to help you embark on an exciting journey toward achieving optimal fitness through the power of aerobics. Whether you are a complete novice or someone looking to refresh your knowledge, this book is your ultimate resource for understanding and mastering the fundamentals of aerobics.

Maintaining a healthy way of life has become more crucial than ever in the fast-paced world of today. Aerobics offers a fun and effective way to improve cardiovascular health, increase endurance, and enhance overall well-being. By engaging in aerobic exercises, you can strengthen your heart, burn calories, and boost your energy levels, all while enjoying the exhilaration of movement.

This book is specifically tailored for beginners, providing step-by-step guidance on how to get started with aerobics and gradually progress toward more advanced levels. We will explore various types of aerobic exercises, including low-impact, high-impact, dance-based, water aerobics, and aerobic circuit training, allowing you to choose the style that best suits your preferences and fitness goals.

To ensure your success, we will delve into essential topics such as warm-up and stretching exercises, proper breathing techniques, designing a personalized workout routine, and incorporating variety into your fitness regimen. Additionally, we will address safety measures, injury prevention, and the importance of nutrition and hydration for optimal performance.

Throughout this book, you will find practical tips, expert advice, and motivational strategies to keep you inspired and focused on your fitness journey. We understand that staying motivated and overcoming challenges can be tough, but with the right mindset and support, you can achieve remarkable results.

Whether your goal is to lose weight, improve cardiovascular health, or simply lead a more active lifestyle, "Aerobics Fitness Guide for Beginners" will equip you with the knowledge and tools necessary to succeed. We believe that fitness should be enjoyable and accessible to everyone, and this book aims to make your aerobics experience both rewarding and fulfilling.

So, are you prepared to make the first move toward a better, healthier version of yourself? Let's dive into the world of aerobics and unlock the incredible benefits it has to offer. Get ready to ignite your passion for fitness, transform your body, and embrace a lifestyle of wellness. The journey starts now.

Chapter 1: Understanding Aerobics: The Basics

1.1 What is Aerobics?

Aerobics, also known as aerobic exercise or cardio, is a form of physical activity that involves rhythmic and continuous movements to increase heart rate and oxygen consumption. It is characterized by exercises that use large muscle groups and can be performed for an extended period. The primary goal of aerobics is to improve cardiovascular fitness, enhance endurance, and burn calories.

1.2 Benefits of Aerobics

Engaging in regular aerobic exercise offers numerous benefits for both the body and mind. It strengthens the heart and lungs, improving their efficiency in delivering oxygen to the muscles. This, in turn, increases overall stamina and endurance. Aerobics also helps to lower blood pressure, reduce the risk of heart disease, and improve cholesterol levels.

Beyond cardiovascular health, aerobics aids in weight management by burning calories and boosting metabolism. It promotes fat loss while preserving lean muscle mass, resulting in a toned and sculpted physique. Additionally, aerobic exercise releases endorphins, known as "feel-good" hormones, which can enhance mood, reduce stress, and alleviate symptoms of anxiety and depression.

1.3 Getting Started: Preparing for Aerobics

Before starting any aerobic exercise program, it is essential to consult with a healthcare professional, especially if you have any underlying medical conditions or concerns. They can provide personalized guidance and ensure that aerobics is safe and suitable for your specific needs.

Once you have the green light, it's time to prepare for your aerobics journey. Start by making attainable goals that support your desire for health.

Whether you aim to lose weight, improve cardiovascular health, or simply increase your energy levels, having a clear objective will help you stay motivated and focused.

Next, consider your current fitness level and choose the appropriate intensity for your workouts. Beginners should start with low to moderate-intensity exercises and gradually increase the duration and difficulty as their fitness improves. It is crucial to listen to your body and avoid pushing yourself beyond your limits to prevent injury.

Furthermore, select the type of aerobic exercise that appeals to you the most. Whether it's dancing, swimming, cycling, or brisk walking, finding an activity that you enjoy will make your workouts more enjoyable and sustainable in the long run.

Lastly, gather the necessary equipment for your aerobics sessions. This may include comfortable workout attire, proper footwear with good cushioning and support, and any additional equipment specific to your chosen aerobic activity.

By taking these initial steps, you are setting the foundation for a successful and fulfilling aerobics journey. In the following chapters, we will delve deeper into the world of aerobics and guide you toward designing a personalized workout routine that suits your needs and preferences. Get ready to experience the incredible benefits of aerobics as we embark on this exciting fitness adventure together.

Chapter 2: Essential Equipment for Aerobics

2.1 Choosing the Right Footwear

When it comes to aerobic exercise, proper footwear is crucial to ensure comfort, support, and injury prevention. The right shoes can enhance your performance and protect your feet from the impact and stress of aerobic movements.

When selecting aerobic shoes, look for the following features:

- **Cushioning:** Adequate cushioning in the midsole and heel helps absorb shock and reduce the risk of impact-related injuries.

- **Arch Support:** Shoes with proper arch support provide stability and help maintain proper alignment during aerobic movements.

- **Breathability:** Look for shoes made from breathable materials to keep your feet cool and dry throughout your workouts.

- **Flexibility:** Shoes with good flexibility allow for natural foot movements and prevent restrictions during aerobic exercises.

- **Traction:** Opt for shoes with a rubber outsole that provides excellent grip and traction on various surfaces.

It is recommended to try on multiple pairs of shoes and walk or jog around the store to ensure a proper fit. Take into consideration the shape and size of your feet, as well as any specific foot conditions or requirements you may have.

2.2 Clothing and Accessories

Choosing the right clothing and accessories for your aerobic workouts can greatly enhance your comfort and performance. **The following are some things to remember:**

- **Moisture-Wicking Fabrics:** Select clothing made from moisture-wicking materials that draw sweat away from your body, keeping you dry and comfortable during intense workouts.

- **Breathable Fabrics:** Opt for breathable fabrics that allow air circulation and prevent overheating.

- **Proper Fit:** Choose clothing that fits well and allows for a full range of motion without being too tight or restrictive.
- **Layering:** Consider layering your clothing to easily adjust to changes in temperature during your workouts.
- **Supportive Sports Bras:** For women, a well-fitting and supportive sports bra is essential to minimize discomfort and provide adequate support during high-impact aerobic activities.
- **Sweatbands and Headbands:** These accessories can help keep sweat out of your eyes and hair during intense workouts.
- **Water Bottle:** Stay hydrated by carrying a water bottle with you during your aerobic sessions.

2.3 Additional Equipment for Aerobic Workouts

Depending on the type of aerobic exercise you choose, there may be additional equipment or props that can enhance your workouts. **Here are a few examples:**
- **Dumbbells or Resistance Bands:** Adding light weights or resistance bands to your aerobic routine

can help increase the intensity and challenge your muscles.

- **Yoga Mat:** If you plan to incorporate floor exercises or stretching into your aerobics routine, a yoga mat can provide cushioning and support.

- **Step Platform:** Step aerobics often requires a step platform, which can be adjusted to different heights to accommodate various fitness levels.

- **Jump Rope:** Jumping rope is a fantastic aerobic exercise that can be done anywhere and provides a great cardiovascular workout.

- **Music and Headphones:** Listening to music can make your aerobic workouts more enjoyable and help you stay motivated. Invest in a good pair of headphones to enhance your listening experience.

Remember, the choice of equipment and accessories will depend on your personal preferences and the type of aerobic exercise you plan to engage in. By selecting the right equipment, you can optimize your aerobic workouts and make them more effective and enjoyable. In the next chapter, we will explore warm-up and stretching exercises to prepare your body for aerobic activities.

Chapter 3: Warm-up and Stretching Exercises

As you embark on your journey into the world of aerobic fitness, it's crucial to understand the pivotal role warm-up and stretching exercises play in ensuring a safe and effective workout session. In this chapter, we delve into the importance of these preparatory steps and provide you with effective techniques to warm up your muscles and stretch your body properly.

3.1 Importance of Warm-up

Before engaging in any physical activity, whether it's a brisk walk or an intense aerobic routine, warming up your muscles is essential. A warm-up serves as a bridge between a state of rest and vigorous exercise. It gradually increases your heart rate, blood flow, and body temperature, preparing your cardiovascular system for the upcoming demands of your workout. Furthermore, a well-executed warm-up enhances your joint mobility, flexibility, and overall athletic performance.

3.2 Effective Stretching Techniques

Stretching is not only a way to enhance flexibility but also a means of preventing injuries. In this section, we'll guide you through various stretching techniques that target different muscle groups. These techniques include static stretching, dynamic stretching, and proprioceptive neuromuscular facilitation (PNF) stretching. We'll also emphasize the importance of holding stretches within your comfort range, avoiding bouncing or jerking movements and breathing steadily during stretches to facilitate relaxation.

3.3 Preparing Your Body for Aerobic Workout

Combining warm-up exercises and stretching forms a holistic approach to preparing your body for the aerobic challenges ahead. We'll provide you with sample warm-up routines that incorporate light

cardiovascular activities such as brisk walking or gentle jogging, gradually elevating your heart rate. Following this, dynamic stretches that mimic the movements of your intended workout can help lubricate your joints and activate specific muscle groups. As we conclude this chapter, you'll have the tools to customize a warm-up and stretching routine that aligns with your unique aerobic workout.

Remember, dedicating time to warming up and stretching not only minimizes the risk of injury but also enhances your overall exercise experience. Your body will thank you for taking these precautionary steps that ultimately contribute to your long-term aerobic fitness goals.

Chapter 4: Different Types of Aerobic Exercises

As you progress in your journey to aerobic fitness, it's essential to explore the variety of exercise options available. This chapter introduces you to the diverse world of aerobic exercises, each offering unique benefits and experiences. Whether you're drawn to high-energy dance routines or prefer the gentle embrace of water workouts, you'll find a style that resonates with your goals and preferences.

4.1 Low-Impact Aerobics

Low-impact aerobic exercises are designed to minimize stress on your joints while still providing an effective cardiovascular workout. These exercises involve at least one foot staying on the ground at all times. This includes riding, swimming, and walking. We'll delve into the benefits of low-impact exercises, which include improving heart health, burning calories, and building endurance without excessive strain on the body.

Benefits of Low-Impact Aerobics: Beyond being joint-friendly, low-impact aerobics offer a host of benefits. We'll explore how these exercises contribute to improved cardiovascular health, increased lung capacity, and enhanced overall endurance. Additionally, the reduced impact makes them an excellent option for individuals recovering from injuries or those looking for a gentler approach to exercise.

Sample Workouts: Dive into sample low-impact workout routines that combine walking, cycling, and swimming. Discover how to structure your sessions to maximize calorie burn and cardiovascular gains while being kind to your joints.

4.2 High-Impact Aerobics

For those seeking a more intense aerobic challenge, high-impact exercises might be the answer. These exercises involve both feet leaving the ground, leading to a higher heart rate and increased calorie burn. Activities like running, jumping jacks, and plyometric exercises fall into this category. We'll guide you through proper techniques and safety considerations to help you embrace the exhilarating world of high-impact workouts.

The Challenge of High-Impact: High-impact aerobic exercises offer a thrilling challenge that pushes your cardiovascular system to new heights. We'll examine how these activities elevate your heart rate rapidly, resulting in increased calorie expenditure and improved cardiovascular fitness.

Safety Precautions: Engaging in high-impact exercises requires attention to proper technique and safety. Learn about essential tips to minimize the risk of injuries, such as wearing appropriate footwear and landing softly to cushion the impact on your joints.

4.3 Dance-Based Aerobics

Dance-based aerobic workouts combine the joy of dancing with the benefits of cardiovascular exercise. From Zumba to hip-hop dance routines, these workouts turn movement into an enjoyable art form. Engaging in dance-based aerobics not only boosts your fitness but also enhances coordination and rhythm. We'll explore different dance styles and provide insights into how to follow choreography even if you're new to dancing.

Beginner-Friendly Approaches: Even if you consider yourself rhythmically challenged, dance-based workouts can be tailored to your abilities. Discover modifications and beginner-friendly routines that allow you to embrace the world of dance aerobics with confidence.

4.4 Water Aerobics

The buoyancy of water offers a unique environment for aerobic exercise. Water aerobics, performed in a pool, provide a low-impact yet challenging workout that's gentle on the joints. The resistance of water increases muscle engagement and adds an extra layer of difficulty to your routine. We'll delve into the benefits of water aerobics and suggest various exercises you can incorporate into your pool workouts.

4.5 Aerobic Circuit Training

Aerobic circuit training combines cardiovascular exercises with strength and resistance training. This multifaceted approach allows you to target both your cardiovascular system and muscular strength in a single workout session. We'll guide you through creating your circuit routines, ensuring a balanced

combination of exercises that elevate your heart rate while also enhancing muscle tone.

By exploring these various types of aerobic exercises, you'll discover a world of options that keep your fitness journey engaging and motivating. Whether you prefer the rhythmic movements of dance or the challenge of high-impact workouts, there's an aerobic exercise style that aligns with your preferences and goals.

Chapter 5: Designing Your Aerobic Workout Routine

Crafting an effective and balanced aerobic workout routine is essential for reaching your fitness goals while ensuring a holistic approach to your well-being. This chapter guides you through the process of structuring a personalized routine that caters to your fitness level, preferences, and aspirations.

5.1 Setting Fitness Goals

• **Defining Your Objectives:** Understand the significance of setting clear and achievable fitness goals. Whether you're aiming for weight loss, improved cardiovascular health, or enhanced endurance, establishing specific objectives provides direction and motivation.

• **SMART Goal Framework:** Learn about the SMART (Specific, Measurable, Achievable, Relevant, Time-bound) criteria for goal-setting. We'll guide you in formulating goals that are well-defined and realistic, ultimately enhancing your commitment to your fitness journey.

5.2 Creating a Balanced Workout Plan

• **Components of a Well-Rounded Routine:** A successful aerobic workout routine encompasses various components beyond cardiovascular exercises. Discover the importance of incorporating strength training, flexibility work, and rest days into your plan.

• **Weekly Frequency and Duration:** Determine how often you should engage in aerobic workouts, considering factors such as your fitness level and schedule. We'll also explore the optimal duration for each session to strike a balance between effectiveness and sustainability.

5.3 Incorporating Variety in Your Routine

• **The Role of Variety:** Preventing workout monotony is crucial for maintaining enthusiasm and progress. Explore the benefits of incorporating diverse aerobic exercises and training methods, ensuring both physical and mental stimulation.

- **Cross-Training Benefits**: Learn how cross-training, or engaging in various types of exercises, can enhance your overall fitness. We'll provide insights into the advantages of alternating between different forms of aerobic workouts.

5.4 Tracking Progress and Making Adjustments

- **The Importance of Monitoring:** Regularly assessing your progress is a key aspect of staying motivated and on track. Discover various methods for tracking your workouts, from maintaining a workout journal to using fitness apps and wearables.
- **Adapting Your Routine:** As your fitness improves, adjustments to your routine become

necessary to continue making progress. We'll guide you through recognizing signs that it's time to increase intensity, change exercises, or modify workout frequency.

By mastering the art of designing a personalized aerobic workout routine, you'll not only optimize your fitness results but also foster a sustainable and enjoyable fitness journey. This chapter equips you with the tools to set meaningful goals, create a balanced plan, embrace variety, and stay adaptable as you progress toward greater aerobic fitness.

Chapter 6: Aerobic Techniques for Beginners

Embarking on an aerobic fitness journey as a beginner requires a solid understanding of foundational techniques. This chapter delves into the fundamental aspects of aerobic exercises, ensuring you're equipped with the knowledge and skills to approach your workouts confidently.

6.1 Basic Steps and Movements

• **Understanding Fundamental Movements:** Explore the basic steps and movements that form the building blocks of aerobic exercises. From marching in place to simple dance steps, we'll break down each movement, allowing you to grasp the essence of aerobic routines.

• **Coordinating Movements with Music:** Learn how to synchronize your movements with music, a hallmark of many aerobic workouts. We'll guide you through the rhythm and timing required to achieve a seamless integration of motion and music.

6.2 Proper Breathing Techniques

- **Breathing and Cardiovascular Efficiency:** Discover how proper breathing techniques enhance the efficiency of your cardiovascular system during aerobic exercises. We'll delve into rhythmic breathing patterns that support sustained effort while preventing overexertion.

- **Incorporating Diaphragmatic Breathing**: Explore diaphragmatic breathing, a technique that promotes deep, efficient breathing by engaging the diaphragm. We'll provide step-by-step instructions to help you practice and implement this beneficial breathing method.

6.3 Intensity and Duration of Workouts

- **Understanding Exercise Intensity:** Grasp the concept of exercise intensity and its impact on your fitness gains. We'll introduce you to methods like the

Rate of Perceived Exertion (RPE) scale, heart rate monitoring, and the Talk Test to gauge and adjust your workout intensity.

• **Gradual Progression:** Avoid the pitfalls of overexertion by learning the art of gradual progression. Discover how to increase the intensity and duration of your workouts at a manageable pace, ensuring consistent improvement without risking injury or burnout.

By immersing yourself in the foundational techniques outlined in this chapter, you'll lay a strong groundwork for your aerobic fitness journey. These techniques, ranging from mastering basic movements to fine-tuning your breathing and understanding workout intensity, empower you to embark on your aerobic exercises with confidence and competence.

Chapter 7: Safety and Injury Prevention in Aerobics

Ensuring your safety and preventing injuries is paramount as you engage in aerobic exercises. This chapter delves into the intricacies of safeguarding your well-being during workouts, equipping you with the knowledge to minimize risks and enjoy a safe and effective fitness journey.

7.1 Understanding Common Aerobic Injuries

- **Identifying Vulnerable Areas:** Explore the parts of the body that are particularly susceptible to injuries during aerobic exercises, such as knees, ankles, and back. Understanding these vulnerabilities is the first step in taking proactive measures.

- **Common Injuries:** We'll delve into common aerobic-related injuries, from sprains and strains to overuse injuries. By recognizing these potential pitfalls, you'll be better equipped to prevent them.

7.2 Preventive Measures and Precautions

• **Proper Warm-up and Cooling Down:** We reiterate the importance of a thorough warm-up and cool-down routine. These practices prepare your muscles and joints for activity and promote recovery after exercise, reducing the likelihood of injury.

• **Form and Technique:** Proper form is a cornerstone of injury prevention. We'll guide you through maintaining correct posture and alignment during exercises, preventing strain on joints and muscles.

7.3 Listening to Your Body: Signs of Overexertion

• **Recognizing Overexertion:** Learn to listen to your body's signals. We'll discuss the signs of overexertion, such as extreme fatigue, dizziness, and shortness of breath, and emphasize the importance of stopping or slowing down when necessary.

• **Rest and Recovery:** Rest days are integral to injury prevention. We'll explore how adequate rest and recovery allow your body to heal and adapt, reducing the risk of chronic injuries.

By embracing the safety measures and injury prevention strategies detailed in this chapter, you'll safeguard your well-being and cultivate a secure environment for your aerobic workouts. The knowledge gained from understanding common injuries, implementing preventive measures, and recognizing overexertion not only protects you but also enhances your ability to fully engage in and enjoy your aerobic fitness journey.

Chapter 8: Nutrition and Hydration for Aerobic Fitness

A successful aerobic fitness journey extends beyond exercise; proper nutrition and hydration play a vital role in achieving your goals. This chapter delves into the significance of fueling your body effectively, providing insights into optimal nutritional choices and hydration practices to maximize your aerobic performance.

8.1 Fueling Your Body for Optimal Performance

• **Balancing Macronutrients:** Understand the importance of a well-balanced diet that incorporates carbohydrates, proteins, and healthy fats. We'll delve into how each macronutrient contributes to sustained energy, muscle repair, and overall vitality.

• **Pre-Workout Nutrition:** Discover the art of pre-workout fueling. Learn when and what to eat before your aerobic session to ensure your body has the necessary energy to perform at its best without causing discomfort.

8.2 Hydration Guidelines for Aerobic Workouts

• **The Significance of Hydration:** Delve into the critical role of hydration in aerobic fitness. We'll explore how staying adequately hydrated improves endurance, aids digestion, and regulates body temperature during exercise.

• **Hydration Timing:** Uncover the best practices for hydrating before, during, and after your workouts. Learn how to gauge your hydration needs based on factors like workout duration and intensity.

8.3 Post-Workout Recovery and Nutrition

• **Recovery Nutrition:** Post-workout nutrition is essential for muscle recovery and replenishing depleted energy stores. We'll discuss the importance of consuming a combination of protein and carbohydrates to promote efficient recovery.

• **Rehydration:** After a workout, rehydrating is equally vital. Learn how to assess your fluid loss and rehydrate appropriately to restore your body's balance.

8.4 Balancing Nutritional Goals and Aerobic Fitness

• **Caloric Needs:** Understand how to adjust your caloric intake to align with your fitness goals, whether you're aiming to lose weight, maintain, or gain muscle. We'll guide you through estimating your energy needs and making informed dietary choices.

• **Nutrient Timing:** Discover the concept of nutrient timing, which involves consuming specific nutrients at optimal times to enhance performance and recovery. This technique ensures that your body receives the right nutrients when it needs them most. By embracing the principles of nutrition and hydration outlined in this chapter, you'll amplify the benefits of your aerobic workouts and accelerate your progress toward your fitness goals. The knowledge gained from understanding macronutrients, mastering pre, and post-workout nutrition, and staying properly hydrated not only fuels your aerobic endeavors but also contributes to your overall health and well-being.

Chapter 9: Motivation and Overcoming Challenges

Maintaining motivation and overcoming challenges are integral components of a successful aerobic fitness journey. This chapter delves into strategies for staying motivated, navigating obstacles, and finding the support needed to ensure your commitment remains steadfast throughout your fitness endeavors.

9.1 Staying Motivated on Your Fitness Journey

• **Setting Short-Term Goals:** Discover the power of setting smaller, achievable goals that contribute to your larger fitness aspirations. These milestones offer a sense of accomplishment, boosting motivation along the way.

• **Visualization Techniques:** Learn the art of visualization, where you mentally picture yourself achieving your fitness goals. Visualization enhances motivation by creating a vivid image of your success, reinforcing your commitment.

9.2 Dealing with Plateaus and Setbacks

• **Understanding Plateaus:** Any fitness journey will inevitably experience plateaus.
 We'll explore why plateaus occur and how to overcome them, whether it's adjusting your routine, intensifying workouts, or seeking variety.

• **Bouncing Back from Setbacks:** Setbacks can be disheartening, but they're not the end of your journey. Learn to view setbacks as opportunities for growth and adapt your approach accordingly.

9.3 Finding Support and Accountability

• **The Role of Support:** Discover the benefits of having a support system, whether it's friends, family, or fellow fitness enthusiasts. Supportive individuals can offer encouragement, share advice, and keep you motivated.

- **Accountability Partners:** Accountability partners provide an extra layer of commitment. We'll delve into the concept of accountability partners and how their presence can significantly enhance your adherence to your fitness routine.

- **Online Communities and Apps:** Explore the wealth of online fitness communities and apps that provide both support and accountability. Engaging with like-minded individuals and tracking your progress electronically can amplify your motivation.

9.4 Mindset and Positive Self-Talk

- **Cultivating a Positive Mindset:** Understand the profound impact of a positive mindset on your fitness journey. Learn how reframing negative thoughts and focusing on your successes can boost your motivation.

- **Harnessing Positive Self-Talk:** Dive into the practice of positive self-talk, where you replace self-criticism with affirmations and encouragement. This technique cultivates self-belief and resilience, crucial for overcoming challenges.

By embracing the motivational strategies and resilience-building techniques detailed in this chapter, you'll cultivate the mental fortitude necessary to conquer obstacles and maintain your commitment to aerobic fitness. The knowledge gained from setting realistic goals, navigating plateaus, seeking support, and fostering a positive mindset not only propels your aerobic journey but also nurtures your personal growth and determination.

Chapter 10: Taking Your Aerobic Fitness to the Next Level

As you grow in your aerobic fitness journey, it's natural to seek new challenges and push your boundaries. This chapter is dedicated to guiding you through the transition from beginner to advanced aerobic exercises, exploring the nuances of higher intensity, diversified routines, and specialized considerations.

10.1 Progressing Beyond Beginner Level

• **Gradual Intensity Increase:** Understand the importance of gradual progression when advancing your aerobic exercises. We'll explore how incremental intensity increases help your body adapt and prevent overexertion.

• **Incorporating Interval Training:** Interval training, alternating between high-intensity bursts and recovery periods, is a powerful technique for advancing your aerobic fitness. Discover how it challenges your cardiovascular system, accelerates calorie burn, and enhances endurance.

10.2 Exploring Advanced Aerobic Workouts

Explore the world of high-intensity interval training (HIIT), a dynamic advanced approach that entails quick bursts of hard activity followed by quick rest intervals.

HIIT maximizes cardiovascular benefits, boosts metabolism, and enhances overall fitness.

Complex Dance Routines: If you've embraced dance-based aerobics, consider delving into more complex dance routines. These advanced routines challenge your coordination, memory, and cardiovascular capacity while offering a joyful and engaging workout.

10.3 Special Considerations for Advanced Training

• **Injury Prevention at Advanced Levels:** As you engage in more intense workouts, injury prevention becomes even more critical. We'll explore how proper form, warm-up routines, and attentive recovery strategies are essential at advanced fitness levels.

• **Nutrition for Advanced Workouts:** Learn how to fine-tune your nutrition to support advanced aerobic training. Discover the optimal macronutrient ratios, supplementation strategies, and recovery foods that cater to the demands of higher-intensity exercises.

10.4 Embracing Periodization

• **Understanding Periodization:** Periodization involves structuring your workouts in cycles of different intensities and focuses. We'll delve into the benefits of periodization, which prevents plateaus, minimizes overtraining, and optimizes performance.

• **Designing Periodized Plans:** Gain insight into creating your periodized aerobic workout plans. We'll guide you through the process of determining

the length of each phase, choosing appropriate exercises, and gradually progressing through the cycles.

By embracing the challenges and strategies outlined in this chapter, you'll elevate your aerobic fitness to new heights, transitioning from beginner to advanced levels with confidence. The knowledge gained from progressing gradually, exploring advanced techniques, considering specialized factors, and implementing periodization not only enhances your physical capabilities but also allows you to enjoy a diverse and fulfilling aerobic fitness journey.

Conclusion

Starting your road to aerobic fitness is a transformative journey that involves your body, mind, and spirit. It is not only a physical endeavor. This guide has illuminated the path from understanding the basics of aerobics to crafting an advanced and personalized fitness regimen. The chapters have been your compass, pointing you toward safety, motivation, and optimal health.

As you stand at the end of this guide, you possess a toolbox overflowing with techniques and wisdom. You comprehend the importance of a warm-up, a fundamental movement, and the grace of breathing in sync with your body's rhythm. You are equipped to prevent injuries and nurture your well-being, knowing when to push and when to pause. You have delved into the art of nutrition and hydration, nourishing not only your physical prowess but your entire being.

Motivation is your ally, and setbacks are stepping stones on this journey. Armed with visualization, support systems, and a positive mindset, you're prepared to conquer the hurdles that come your way.

The plateau is but temporary, a mere chapter in your story of progress and achievement.

As you traverse from a novice to a seasoned practitioner, you have unlocked the secrets of advanced workouts. High-intensity intervals and complex dance routines are your playgrounds, driven by a foundation of knowledge in periodization and tailored nutrition. With each workout, you sculpt your body and spirit, embracing the rhythm of discipline and growth.

Remember, this journey isn't just about the destination; it's about the transformation that occurs along the way. The sweat, the sore muscles, and the sense of accomplishment are all part of the tapestry you weave, a testament to your dedication and perseverance. This guide has provided you with a map, but the landscape you traverse is uniquely yours.

As you move forward, let this guide be your companion, a reference in times of need, and a reminder of the power within you. Your aerobic fitness journey is a symphony of movement, a dance of dedication, and a celebration of the human spirit's capability for change. The culmination of understanding, practice, and commitment is the symphony's crescendo. You are the conductor, and the journey is your masterpiece.

Believe in yourself because you have the ability to change your life and your body. With each step, each movement, and each breath, embrace the journey of aerobics and discover the strength within. Remember, every beginner was once a beginner, and every expert started with a single step. So, let your determination ignite, your dedication shine, and your passion soar as you embark on this empowering path of aerobics body fitness. You are capable, you are resilient, and you are destined for greatness. Embrace the challenge, embrace the sweat, and embrace the joy of becoming the best version of yourself. Let your journey inspire others, as you inspire yourself. Believe in the power of aerobics, and let your body and spirit soar to new heights. You've got this!"

Appendix: Sample Aerobic Workout Routines

In the spirit of practicality, this appendix presents a collection of sample aerobic workout routines tailored to different fitness levels and goals. These routines serve as templates to guide you in structuring your own effective and diverse workouts. Feel free to modify and customize them according to your preferences, needs, and progress.

Beginner's Routine: Cardio Kickstart

- 5 minutes of vigorous walking or light jogging serve as a warm-up.
- Low-Impact Aerobics: 20 minutes of alternating between marching in place, step taps, and knee lifts.
- Strength Training: 10 minutes of bodyweight exercises like squats, lunges, and push-ups.
- Cool-down: 5-10 minutes of gentle stretches for major muscle groups.

• *Intermediate Routine: Dance Fusion*

- Warm-up: 5-7 minutes of light cardio, such as jumping jacks or jogging in place.
- Dance-Based Aerobics: 25-30 minutes of following a choreographed dance routine incorporating various dance styles.
- High-Intensity Intervals: 10 minutes of alternating between 30 seconds of high-intensity moves (burpees, mountain climbers) and 30 seconds of rest.
- Core Strengthening: 10 minutes of exercises like planks, Russian twists, and bicycle crunches.
- Cool-down: 5-10 minutes of static stretches for flexibility.

• *Advanced Routine: Total Body HIIT*

- Warm-up: 7-10 minutes of dynamic stretches and light cardio (skipping, leg swings).
- High-Intensity Interval Training (HIIT): 20-25 minutes of alternating between 45 seconds of high-intensity exercises (sprints, jump squats) and 15 seconds of rest.
- Circuit Strength Training: 15-20 minutes of 3 circuits, each including 3 strength exercises targeting different muscle groups.

- Complex Dance Routine: 10-15 minutes of a challenging dance routine incorporating intricate steps and transitions.
- Cool-down: 10 minutes of deep stretches for relaxation and recovery.

These sample routines are mere starting points, illustrating how you can structure your workouts to achieve specific goals. Remember, safety and personalization are paramount. Listen to your body, progress gradually, and adjust exercises as needed. With dedication and consistency, these routines will serve as your foundation for creating unique and impactful aerobic workouts that propel you toward your fitness aspirations.

www.ingramcontent.com/pod-product-compliance
Lightning Source LLC
Chambersburg PA
CBHW070733260726

48660CB00007B/2821